Activities for the Family Caregiver

MULTIPLE SCLEROSIS

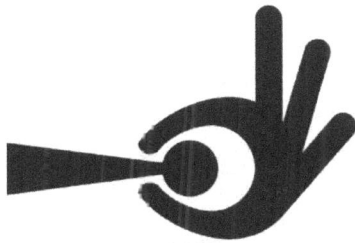

R.O.S.

HOW TO ENGAGE
HOW TO LIVE

Scott Silknitter, Suzanne John, RN
Lisa Ost-Beikmann, ADC, CDP, AC-BC,
CADDCT, CAEd

Disclaimer

This book is for informational purposes only and is not intended as medical advice, diagnosis, or treatment. Always seek advice from a qualified physician about medical concerns, and do not disregard medical advice because of something you may read within this book. This book does not replace the need for diagnostic evaluation, ongoing physician care, and professional assessment of treatments. Every effort has been made to make this book as complete and helpful as possible. It is important, however, for this book to be used as a resource and idea-generating guide and not as an ultimate source for plan of care.

ISBN 978-1-943285-21-1

Published by
R.O.S. Therapy Systems, L.L.C.
Greensboro, NC
888-352-9788
www.ROSTherapySystems.com

Table of Contents

Family Members and Caregivers
that have read this book:

_____

_____

_____

_____

_____

_____

_____

_____

_____

_____

_____

Chapter 1

MS Overview and Symptoms

Multiple sclerosis (MS) affects millions of people around the world. With MS, the nerves of the brain and spinal cord are damaged by one's own immune system.

Although the disease was discovered in 1868, the cause of MS largely remains a mystery. We know that the nerve damage is due to inflammation, but the exact cause of the inflammation is still unknown.

MS is a progressive, "immune-mediated" disease. This means that the body system designed to keep us healthy mistakenly attacks parts of the body that are vital to everyday function. During these "attacks," protective coverings of nerve cells are damaged leading to diminished brain and spinal cord function.

The nerve cell damage leads to symptoms, which can range from mild to severe in intensity. The progress and specific symptoms are unpredictable. While some people experience mild issues, such as fatigue, other people may experience more severe issues, such as paralysis, vision loss, and chronic pain.

If your loved one is experiencing a single symptom or multiple symptoms of MS, it can have a dramatic effect on their quality of life and yours. Our goal is to help your loved one engage in activities and to provide tips and tools to help you and your loved one maintain quality of life.

Let's take a deeper look at many of the symptoms your loved one could experience.

Tingling and Numbness

Numbness of the arms and legs, face, or body is often one of the first symptoms of MS. As discussed, MS affects nerves within the brain and spinal cord. This means that conflicting signals or no signals at all may be sent around the body, which can result in tingling and numbness. When this happens, it will affect your loved one's ability to engage in standard daily activities.

Fatigue

Fatigue occurs when nerves deteriorate within the spinal column. The fatigue appears suddenly and can last for weeks before improving. The fatigue can significantly interfere with the ability to function at home and at work.

Visual Impairments

Vision impairments are one of the most common symptoms suffered by someone with MS. Blurred vision, poor contrast or color vision, and painful eye movement are all items that your loved one may experience. Your loved one may not notice the vision issues right away, as the degeneration of clear vision can be slow.

A loved one who is visually impaired adds another element for which their caregiver should be mindful. For successful interactions with a visually impaired person, preparation is key. As caregiving is a 24/7 job, so is the preparation of everything in your loved one's life. From the time they wake up, to the time they go to bed, from getting dressed, or eating a meal, everything must be prepared. Like all of us, our loved ones are individuals with their own wants, likes, needs, and preferences. As caregivers, we need to ensure that we are setting them up for success. Areas to focus for that preparation include:

- Organization
- Lighting and Glare
- Contrast

Weakness

Weakness is a result from damage to nerves that stimulate muscles or deconditioning of unused muscles. This will affect your loved one's ability to engage in active activities, such as walking, tai chi, dancing, or yoga. Those activities are also items that can be a part of a rehabilitation program should your loved one's therapist approve and recommend.

Pain

Chronic or significant pain is common with MS. One study through the National Multiple Sclerosis Society showed that half of people with MS experience pain.

Walking and Balance Problems

Your loved one may experience trouble walking related to several factors, such as weakness, spasticity, loss of balance, sensory deficit, and fatigue. Your loved one's doctor may refer to these as problems with their gait.

Dizziness

Your loved one may feel lightheaded, dizzy, or as if their surroundings are spinning (vertigo). This symptom often occurs when a person stands up.

Stiffness and Muscle Spasms

Spasticity refers to feelings of stiffness and a wide range of involuntary muscle spasms. This can happen in any of your loved one's limbs.

Bladder and Bowel Problems

Bladder problems can dramatically affect your loved one's sense of well-being and ability to "do things." Why? If your loved one is experiencing frequent urination, strong urges to urinate, or inability to hold in urine, they may be more focused on being closer to a bathroom than engaging in any activities. They may pass on outings or other activities with friends and families if they feel like they are going to spend all of their time trying to find or visiting a bathroom.

The same can be said for bowel problems. They may happen less often for someone with MS, but your loved one may experience constipation, diarrhea, or loss of bowel control.

Sexual Problems

Sexual problems and arousal may be a problem for your loved one. Damage to the central nervous system caused by MS is a cause, along with other MS symptoms, such as fatigue, pain, or spasticity.

Cognitive Problems

About half of the people with MS develop some type of issue with their cognitive function. This can include:

- Memory problems
- Shortened attention span
- Language problems
- Difficulty staying organized

Emotional Health

Major depression and/or other emotional health problems can be common among those diagnosed with MS. The stresses of MS may lead to irritability, mood swings, and uncontrollable crying and laughing.

Coping with MS symptoms is difficult enough, but when you add in relationship or family issues, it can make depression and other emotional disorders even more challenging.

Other Symptoms

MS affects everyone differently. Not everyone will have the same individual or combination of symptoms, and occasionally, symptoms can vary in the same person. In addition to the symptoms listed above, other symptoms that may affect your loved one during relapses or attacks include:

- Speech problems
- Tremors
- Hearing loss
- Seizures
- Breathing problems
- Trouble swallowing
- Headaches

Progression and Severity

Attacks can last a few weeks and then disappear. Relapses may get progressively worse and more unpredictable. Early detection and preparation are key for you and your loved one to maintain as high a quality of life as possible during attacks and relapses. Please note that much of the information and preparation tools may not seem necessary if your loved one is feeling fine, but when an attack happens, you will be able to use the information in this book to engage your loved one.

Chapter 2

Activities, Their Benefits, and the Family

"Activities" and "Activities of Daily Living" (ADLs) are critical aspects to caring for your loved one at home. Both types, leisure and daily living, require knowledge of your loved one's habits, preferences, abilities, and routines. This knowledge will enhance the ability of all caregivers to communicate and execute a planned activity with your loved one. Life happens, and things can happen spontaneously, but all activities should be planned to offer the best possible outcome to enhance your loved one's sense of well-being and to promote or enhance their physical, cognitive, and emotional health. In this book, we will focus on leisure activities and the activities of daily living with common sense suggestions and tips on the "How To's" of getting your loved one engaged, dressed, or fed.

In the institutional setting of today, Leisure Activities are required by law if a nursing home accepts government funding. In these situations, Activities are to be provided to every resident on a daily basis based on an individual's preferences. Activities has grown into a profession where Certified Activity Professionals and their staff plan and execute leisure activity programs for residents and seniors in their care.

In addition, professional staff members are required to undergo annual training on the basics of Activities of Daily Living in order to provide better care for the residents they work with. There is plenty of support for professional caregivers to engage people in activities in facilities, but it can be a challenge for caregivers to do the same, important work for loved ones in the home.

Given that there are millions of families and informal caregivers who care for their loved ones with MS at home, it is very important

that some of the pertinent skills and
training of formal, certified caregivers are
made accessible.

Recognizing the growth in the numbers of
those caring for a loved one at home due to
financial need or a simple desire to just be at
home, the R.O.S. Engagement Program and
this book are based on the principles and
approaches used by professionals to assist
with the daily living activities of those with
MS. This was done for two reasons.

1. Provide family caregivers the knowledge
   and tools to allow them to engage their
   loved one so that both can enjoy the
   benefits of activities.

2. Offer a starting point that will provide
   continuity of approach regarding care,
   communication, and information-gathering
   to minimize changes and acclimation time
   if your loved one does have to move from
   home to an institutional setting.

If you choose to use the services of a home care agency while caring for your loved one at home, please ask if they have a Home Care Certified professional on staff, and make sure that the caregiver you choose has received basic training on Leisure Activities and Activities of Daily Living. This will assist with continuity of approach, communication, and planning that will benefit both you and your loved one.

Our goal is to help you deliver meaningful programs of interest to your loved one that focus on physical, social, spiritual, cognitive, and recreational activities. Everyone involved in the care for your loved one should be "on the same page" to minimize changes and challenges that your loved one will face.

Not all family members may understand or accept your loved one's MS. Your loved one may look the same on the outside and may be having a "good day" when someone comes to visit. Family members who visit occasionally may not understand or see all of the symptoms that primary caregivers see daily. They may underestimate or minimize the responsibilities or stress of being a caregiver. This can create conflict. If it helps to avoid a conflict or stress, please have the family members read this book prior to a visit, so they can begin to understand the monumental task that you face as a caregiver. Use visits and interactions as teaching moments.

It can take a while to learn new roles and responsibilities. It is critical, however, to have as many family members and friends involved in your loved one's life as possible. This is not just to show your loved one they are cared for and loved, but also to give you, the primary family caregiver, the occasional and much-needed break.

The importance of understanding your family dynamics and the role each individual plays in the family will lead to better understanding and comprehension for the future. As the MS progresses, roles will evolve, and everyone needs to understand that.

Whether family members come for an occasional visit or visit regularly every week, each one can play an important role in your loved one's life. Family members can help with caregiving, preparing the home to ensure safety and quality of life, and successfully engaging with the loved one you care for.

The Benefits of Activities with a Standard Approach

Caregiver Benefits

Planned and well-executed activities result in less stress for the caregiver as well as less stress for your loved one. Whether it is playing a game or bathing, a standard approach where as many details are planned as possible, can make a significant, positive difference for everyone.

Social Benefits of Activities

Activities offer the opportunity for increased social interaction between family members, friends, caregivers, and the one being cared for. Activities create positive experiences and memories for everyone.

Behavioral Benefits of Activities

Well-planned and well-executed activities of any type can reduce challenging behaviors that sometimes arise when caring for someone with cognitive deficits.

Self-Esteem Benefits of Activities

Leisure activities offered at the right skill level provide your loved one with an opportunity for success. This is also true with Activities of Daily Living, such as dressing. Success during activities improves how your loved one feels about themselves.

Sleep Benefits of Activities

As part of a daily routine, activities can improve sleeping at night. If a loved one is inactive all day, it is likely they will nap periodically. Napping can interrupt good sleep patterns at night.

Being a primary caregiver is a 24/7 job. Without help, you are always on call and run the risk of becoming physically and mentally exhausted.

When you do bring in help, make sure all of your loved one's caregivers (full-time, part-time, family and friends) use the same approach for activities and interaction that you do. With a common approach, there are significantly less opportunities to disrupt routines and make unsettling changes that affect you and your loved one long after the help has left.

A common approach is key. Demand it!

The Four Pillars of Activities

The R.O.S. Engagement Pram focuses on the Four Pillars of Activities. These are areas that all caregivers for your loved one should be familiar with to provide continuity of care and give your loved one the greatest opportunity for success to engage and improve the quality of life for everyone.

First Pillar of Activities: Know your Loved One—Information Gathering and Assessment

Have a Personal History Form completed. Know them—who they are, who they were, and what their functional abilities are today. Make sure all caregivers know this as well.

Second Pillar of Activities: Communicating and Motivating for Success

Communication is key. Each caregiver must know how to effectively communicate with your loved one and be consistent with techniques.

Third Pillar of Activities: Customary Routines and Preferences

As best as possible, maintain a routine and daily plan based on your loved one's needs and preferences.

Fourth Pillar of Activities: Planning and Executing Activities

Based on all of the information you have gathered about your loved one, you have the opportunity to offer engaging activities that are appropriate and meet your loved one's personal preferences.

Chapter 3

First Pillar of Activities:
Know Your Loved One—
Information Gathering
and Assessment

It is important, before you begin providing personal care, that you first recognize various personal attributes and abilities of your loved one and yourself. The more you know about your loved one's lifestyle, likes, and dislikes, the easier providing for their personal and leisure needs will be.

Make it your goal as a caregiver to make available their past interests so they can continue to enjoy them as well as be reminded of previous "good times" they shared with family and friends.

Knowing your loved one is the First Pillar of Activities. Knowing their individual needs, interests, and capabilities will assist you in knowing how to communicate with them and plan or engage in activities with them.

It is important to concentrate on what your loved one **_CAN DO_**, not on what they **_CANNOT DO_**. You must look at everything. Can they pick up a fork and feed themselves; can they get in and out of the bathtub on their own; can they still see the daily crossword in the newspaper that they have enjoyed for years? Big things and little things—they all matter. Details are critical and as you focus on the things that your loved one can do and enjoy, you can plan and execute activities so everyone sees the benefits of activities listed earlier in this book. Therefore, the more you know about your loved one, the more effective you can be as a caregiver. Caregiving routines should be kept structured and regular.

As a caregiver, you will need to provide both the support and the resources to allow your loved one to maintain physical activities to their best ability. You probably already know this, but you are a superhero, a cheerleader, a nurse, a cook, a friend, a protector, a therapist, and much more to your loved one. The more you know and remember about your loved one, the better opportunities you have to connect in order to continue to be that superhero, especially during and after an attack.

You and your loved one may have been very private people. Having MS may change that. Gathering information and sharing with other caregivers is critical as your loved one's past pleasures, likes, and activities will become cornerstones of the communication process for everyone.

If there is something that you might consider embarrassing or private and choose not to share what happened years ago, please note that one way or another, it will come out.

Whatever it was that you think is difficult to share, caregivers and family members that offer assistance are not there to judge you or your loved one on something that happened years or even decades ago. They are there to help you in your moment of need today. Knowing your loved one is vital to the communication process and allows all caregivers the opportunity to turn a "bad" day into a "good" day through proper communication techniques.

As the primary caregiver, you may already know most of the answers, but this is a good and necessary exercise for you, other family members, and other caregivers to execute. We suggest everyone fill out the Personal History Form at the back of this book, but as a starting point, you, the primary caregiver, are most likely able to provide the following basic information:

Basic Information

Name, preferred name to be called, age, and date of birth

Background Information

Place of birth, cultural/ethnic background, marital status, children (how many, and their names), religion/church, military service/employment, education level, and primary language spoken

Medical and Dietary/Nutritional Information

Any formal diagnosis, allergies, and food regimen/diets

Habits

Drinking/alcohol, smoking, exercise, and other things that are a daily habit

Physical Status

Abilities/limitations, visual aids, hearing deficits, speech, communication, hand dominance, and mobility/gait

Mental Status

Alertness; cognitive abilities/limitations; orientation to family, time, place, person, routine; ability to follow directions; preference for written or verbal instructions; ability to comprehend and follow one-step versus multi-step directions; safety awareness; safety concerns; etc.

Social Status

One-on-one interaction; being visited; communication with others through written words, phone calls, or other means, such as email or online social networking services

Emotional Status

Level of contentment, outgoing/withdrawn, extroverted/introverted, dependent/independent, easily frustrated, easygoing

Leisure Status

Past, present, and possible future interests; solitary versus social activities; physical versus passive activities

Vision Status

Any impairment they may have

Informal Assessments

Informal assessments are done through interviews, observation, and information gathered through other means. These will allow you and others to "fill in the blanks" of the Personal History Form.

Interviews

Interviews are conducted with your loved one, or with family members, friends, or significant others.

Observation

An observation is what you and others have seen or heard concerning your loved one, e.g., how they interact with others, their behavior, and their responses to questions or statements made by others. This includes body language and expressions. You have probably seen these interactions a thousand times and made a mental note whenever something stuck out. Now, you must write them down for your future use and for others.

Assessment Tips for Visual Impairment

- Everyone's vision impairment is very different. Assessments and activities must be based on your loved one's remaining vision strength. Some people who are legally blind function very independently. Others may have significant vision loss allowing them to only see shadows or light perception.

- As each vision impairment differs, so does the individual's reactions, feelings, abilities, and needs. The individual assessment will provide necessary information to provide meaningful activities.

- The assessment function is an ongoing function. As the visual or cognitive impairment of your loved one progresses, all caregivers must contribute to keep the information up to date and relevant to ensure consistency in approach or cues when engaging your loved one in an activity.

Information Gathered Through Other Means

Make a request of family members or friends to help complete the Personal History Form at the back of this book. You also may download a copy of the Personal History Form at www.StartSomeJoy.org. Gather as much information as possible and share it with all caregivers—family, informal, and formal.

Your ability to identify past preferences is vital to the planning and execution of an activity, which we will cover in this book. Details matter.

Let's look at someone who enjoys gardening.

During their assessments, three people might all say they like "working in the garden/house plants," yet they might not actually have the same activity in mind.

- Person 1—Enjoys planting and caring for roses on a regular basis then will cut them back and place them in vases to give as gifts or decorate the table.

- Person 2—Enjoys annual flowers that can be changed out and rearranged in the garden each year.

- Person 3—Enjoys working with varieties of green plants that can be trimmed back and rooted to start new plants for family and friends.

As you can see from these examples, details matter. Gather as much information as you can for yourself and all caregivers who may help with your loved one.

Chapter 4

Second Pillar of Activities: Communicating and Motivating for Success

Communicating and motivating for success is the Second Pillar for engaging in an activity with your loved one. The key to effective communication is the ability to listen attentively. This requires all caregivers to use communication techniques that provide an open, nonthreatening environment for your loved one. Listening behavior can either enhance and encourage communication or shut down communication altogether. You need to assess your listening style and be able to assess the listening styles of the other caregivers and family members working with your loved one.

Verbal Communication

Communication is simply an interactive process whereby information is exchanged. More importantly, though, communication is a way to connect with another person. How well you connect depends on your ability to respond appropriately and give feedback on something that was communicated. It also depends on your ability to ***listen***.

Verbal Approaches for Good Communication

- Use exact, short, positive phrases. Repeat twice if necessary.

- Speak slowly with words your loved one knows.

- Allow time for your loved one to answer. Avoid finishing others' sentences.

- Give one instruction at a time. Provide only the number of steps your loved one can handle at a time.

- Use a friendly, respectful tone of voice.

- There is no need to shout, unless your loved one also has a hearing impairment.

- If your loved one is unable to see you because of a visual impairment, be sure to use verbal cues to let them know you are engaged.

- Talk to your loved one like an adult.

Verbal Communication Tips

- Make your presence known when entering a room by saying hello.

- If there are others present, address your loved one by name so there is no confusion as to whom you are speaking.

- Indicate the end of a conversation with a loved one who is totally blind or severely visually impaired to avoid the embarrassment of leaving your loved one speaking when no one is actually there.

- Speak directly to your loved one.

- Always answer questions, and be specific in your responses.

- When giving directions, make the directions as clear as possible. Use "left" and "right" according to the way your loved one is facing.

- Provide a written summary of information/instructions as needed if memory is an issue.

- When speaking with other caregivers or family members about your loved one while they are present, make sure the conversation is respectful of your loved one, and be sure to include your loved one in the conversation to avoid it being "about" them.

- Avoid battles or direct confrontations. For example, avoid situations wherein you are telling someone to do something.

Nonverbal Communication

Although it may seem that most communication happens verbally, research has shown that actually most communication occurs nonverbally. Nonverbal communication occurs through an individual's body language. It can go a long way to convey your message and make your connection stronger, but it can also undercut your attempts to communicate if your nonverbal cues contradict your intention or send mixed signals. Even if your loved one is experiencing vision loss due to MS, your efforts to communicate positively through nonverbal cues and signals do matter.

The key elements to consider regarding how you communicate nonverbally include:

Facial Expressions

Be aware of what your facial expressions are conveying to your loved one. Your mood will be mirrored.

Eye Contact

Ensure that you have made eye contact with your loved one and that their attention is focused on you and what you are saying.

Gestures and Touch

Calmly use nonverbal signs, such as pointing, waving, and other hand gestures in combination with your words.

Tone of Voice

The inflection in your voice helps your loved one relate to the words you are saying.

Body Language

Be aware of the position of your hands and arms when talking to your loved one.

*Note: When communicating with your loved one, be mindful that their body language may not fully tell how they feel or what they are trying to express because of MS. Your body language, however, will be read by your loved one.

Nonverbal Communication Tips

- Always approach your loved one from the front before speaking to them.

- Smile and extend your hand as to shake their hand. Use touch where welcomed.

- Do not touch unexpectedly; it might startle your loved one.

- Place yourself at eye level with the loved one with whom you are speaking.

- Use nonverbal gestures along with words.

- Give nonverbal praises, such as smiles and head nods.

- Be an active listener. Give your loved one opportunities and time to speak. If your loved one has a visual impairment, they may not necessarily see the look of interest on your face, so give verbal cues to let them know that you are actively listening.

- Make sure that all caregivers give your loved one the opportunity and time to speak.

- If you need to make direct contact with your loved one, announce what is about to take place.

- If your loved one has a visual impairment, make eye contact and face the person with whom you are speaking. Provide them the same courtesy you would a person without a visual impairment.

Being a Detective

If your loved one is having an attack, you may not know what the day is going to hold—or even if it will be a good day or a bad day. This is because symptoms can vary each time. If there is an issue, the starting point in your process is communicating to figure out what they are telling you.

Approaches to Successful Communication

Be Calm

Always approach your loved one in a relaxed and calm demeanor. Remember, your mood will be mirrored by your loved one. Smiles are contagious.

Be Flexible

There is no right or wrong way of completing a task. Offer praise and encouragement for the effort your loved one puts into a task. If you see your loved one becoming overwhelmed or frustrated, stop the task, and re-approach at another time.

Be Nonresistive

Do not force tasks on your loved one. Adults do not want to be told, "No!" or told what to do. The power of suggestion goes a long way, and you get more with an ounce of sugar than you do a pound of vinegar.

Be Guiding, but Not Controlling

Always use a soft, gentle approach, and remember your tone of voice. Your facial expressions must match the words you are saying.

These guidelines are effective and should be followed by you and all family members or other caregivers of your loved one. Let's look at an example of how a common approach by all caregivers can be effective in creating a positive day.

Your loved one's favorite game is Scrabble, and the two of you have played it on a regular basis for years. He would set up the game as you set out the coffee and cookies to share. Due to him being a college professor, he was always confident in winning, but the two of you together made it "fun." Previously, he was able to do everything the same—just at a slower place.

As the disease has progressed, your loved one is slower with the words, and you are now helping him write the score as it becomes frustrating for him. Your family has purchased the Scrabble swivel game board, which the letters "lock" into, and it is a great relief to him.

You have become worn out with your loved one's frustration and occasional anger. You do not quite know how to help without doing it for him, and that is the last thing he wants. One day while sharing your concerns with your two children, they come up with an idea to share the load with their children. Their boys love their grandfather dearly and eagerly accept the idea to be his "partner" in the game.

So, the following week the grandsons offer to assist and take turns with their grandfather in a Scrabble game. He is thrilled with their attention and is genuinely pleased that they will handle the small letters so he does not have to. The family time is just as important as the intellectual time, and dad enjoys everyone around the dining room table. It becomes a bi-weekly event, and you have time to rest or do other things you enjoy.

During the final stages when Dad/Grandpa cannot communicate, his grandson picks a word and gets a "yes" or "no" nod from Grandpa before playing.

Planning, patience, effective communication, and the ability to adapt are all easier said than done if you are in the heat of the moment where everything that could happen, does happen.

Armed with the knowledge of your loved one's past, and effective communication skills, all caregivers have the opportunity to engage your loved one in a meaningful activity that will improve the quality of your loved one's life and theirs.

Please remember that your loved one did not choose to be here. If they could choose not to have MS, they would not have it. You must use all of the resources available to you, such as this book, to be ready when it does happen. Accept help when it is offered, and take time to take care of yourself whenever the opportunity arises. As much as it may feel like it at certain times, you are not alone in this fight.

Barriers to Good Communication

Caregiver barriers and environmental barriers can negatively affect communication with your loved one. Here are some tips on how to eliminate these two barriers.

Caregiver Barriers to Communication

Make sure that everyone, including you and anyone that comes in to assist your loved one, is on the same page and use the same verbal communication approaches. Here are some items to avoid:

- Do not speak too quickly. Slow down and speak clearly.

- Do not raise your voice. Use a calm tone, and be aware of your hand movements.

- Never be demanding or commanding.

- Do not offer long explanations when answering questions.

- Do not let your anger and frustration at various situations build and turn into hurtful words.

Environmental Barriers to Communication

With so many things happening around us, we must make sure to remove, or adapt to, avoidable communication barriers around us. Here are some examples:

- Barking dogs can make it a challenge to speak with your loved one. If you can wait until the barking stops, or shush the dogs before speaking to you loved one, this will help.

- Minimize noise from air conditioners and home appliances.

- Running water from a kitchen sink or bathtub can be an issue. Try to wrap up a conversation before the water is turned on. If your loved one is trying to speak while the water is running, turn the water off.

- Turn off the TV if it is on in the same room where you are trying to talk.

- Be aware of outside traffic noise.

- Adjust the lighting in the room. If the lighting in a room makes seeing even more difficult for someone with limited vision, they may be more focused on trying to see rather than on communicating with you.

Barriers of any type will have a negative effect on communication and could possibly lead to a behavioral issue if your loved one thinks you are yelling at them for no particular reason even though you were only trying to be loud enough for them to hear you. Here is an example of something you can try. You have been trying to have a conversation with your loved one. You are making eye contact and standing directly in front of them, but you are still having trouble connecting because the TV is playing in the background, and the dogs are barking at the door.

There are three things happening at the same time: your attempt at conversation, the television, and the barking dogs. This can be very overstimulating for your loved one, and they do not know where to focus. A good idea would be to address the needs of the dogs, and then as you walk into the room smiling, go turn the volume of the television down, or turn it off completely, while you explain you have a question to ask. You can then sit down at eye level with your loved one before speaking.

Communication, Behaviors, and Frustration

Behaviors are a means to communicate when words are not effective.

Caregivers must uncover the meaning behind the behaviors and put a plan into effect to manage those needs. Be a detective.

Aggressive Behaviors

Aggressive behaviors can be defined as hitting, angry outbursts, obscenities, yelling, racial insults, making inappropriate sexual comments and/or biting. Trying to communicate with, or provide care to, a person who is aggressive can be stressful and even frightening for caregivers.

For example, you are engaging in activity with your loved one, and everything is going well. Suddenly, out of nowhere your loved one becomes very angry. They begin using profanity while telling you to get out and leave them alone. A good approach would be to validate their feelings and behavior with a simple and calmly spoken comment/question while you are trying to figure out the cause.

"Roger, you seem very angry today. What are you angry about?"

Based on clues presented, you may discover that your loved one feels helpless and is angry about his loss of abilities. This is an opportunity to further validate their feelings and direct the focus to the positives of remaining abilities they do have.

You may have to stop what you were trying to do with your loved one and just focus on their feelings. You may need to give them space and retry the task another time.

Each situation will be unique and you must work through the issues one at a time.

Possible Causes for Aggression

- Too much noise or overstimulation
- Cluttered environment
- Uncomfortable room temperatures
- Basic needs not being met: hunger, thirst, needing to use the bathroom, needing comfort
- Pain
- Fear, anxiety, or confusion
- Communication barriers
- Frustration at their situation

- Caregiver's mood

- Feeling that they are being rushed

- Difficulty seeing activity or materials of activity, which prevents them from participating

- Lack of independence

<u>Interventions to Utilize</u>
<u>to Mitigate Aggressive Behaviors</u>

- Validate and support their feelings.

- Reminisce with your loved one about specific details of their past.

- Remain calm, and speak in a soft tone.

- Find items that they find comfort in, e.g., a picture of the family.

- Provide consistent caregivers and schedules. Stick to your loved one's routine.

- Engage in recreational activities that match their abilities and interests, as tolerated.

- Break down instructions into one-step increments.

- Identify the triggers of the aggression. Be a detective. There is never a behavior that just occurs.

- Keep an ongoing dialogue between family members and caregivers over any noted changes in patterns or behaviors.

- Help your loved one to slow down and relax.

- Play or listen to music your loved one enjoys for its calming effects.

- Use spiritual support if this is important to your loved one.

Chapter 5

Third Pillar of Activities:
Customary Routines and Preferences

Customary routines and preferences is the Third Pillar in an activities program. Activities can occur all day, every day. The question should not be, "When should I do activities?" It is not important to focus on when to do activities. The focus should be on making each and every interaction that is a part of your loved one's daily routine memorable and enjoyable.

For the purpose of developing a daily plan of care, we will be discussing two areas: Daily Customary Routine and Activity Preferences. The goal is to gain from your loved one's perspective how important certain aspects of care/activity are of interest to them as an individual.

Daily Customary Routine

Your loved one has distinct lifestyle preferences and routines. They should be preserved to the greatest extent possible. All reasonable accommodation should be made to maintain their lifestyle preferences.

Not accommodating your loved one's lifestyle preferences and routine can contribute to a depressed mood and increased behavior symptoms. When a person feels like their control has been removed and that their preferences are not respected as an individual, it can be demoralizing.

Activity Preferences

Activities are a way for individuals to establish meaning in their lives. The need for enjoyable activities does not change based on their age or health needs. The only thing that changes is the level of assistance they may need to engage in those pursuits.

A lack of opportunity to engage in meaningful and enjoyable activities can result in boredom, depression, and behavioral disturbances.

Individuals vary in the activities they prefer, reflecting unique personalities, past interest, perceived environmental constraints, religious and cultural background, and changing physical and mental abilities. We as family caregivers have a great opportunity to empower a loved one to see that they possess many great talents and abilities. By modifying or adapting an activity to allow them to engage at an independent level, you are restoring their self-esteem and self-worth.

Chapter 6

Fourth Pillar of Activities: Planning and Executing Activities

Planning and executing activities is the Fourth Pillar in engaging a loved one in an activity. With the knowledge of your loved one's history, effective communication techniques to use, and their daily routine, we now look at planning activities in which they can be successful.

The Lesson Plan

The Lesson Plan template is a guideline for an activity. Each loved one's abilities and responses are different. This will dictate how you modify an activity to meet their individual needs and abilities. The Lesson Plan is an ever-changing document. It is meant to be written on to note any changes needed so the next person working with your loved one can follow your modifications in hopes of recreating a positive experience.

Items in the Lesson Plan

Date

Document the date the activity is used with your loved one.

Activity Name

Give the activity a name that you or your loved one prefers.

Objective of Activity

Our goal is to provide meaningful activities. People have a need to be productive, and they want to engage in something with a purpose. List the objectives of the program.

Materials

List of suggested materials to use with this activity.

Prerequisite Skills

The skills your loved one needs to participate in this activity.

Activity Outline

Step-by-step instructions to complete
this activity.

Evaluation

When you or a family member are conducting
an activity with your loved one, documenting
results and responses is critical to identifying
ways to improve activity programs for your
loved one. Items to document should include:

- Verbal cues, physical assistance, or
  modifications you make to activity.

- How your loved one responded to
  this activity.

- Did your loved one enjoy this activity
  or not?

- Was the activity successful at distracting
  or eliminating a negative behavior?

A blank template is included on the next page
to give you an example of what a Lesson Plan
looks like.

Lesson Plan Blank Example

Date	Activity Name

Objective of Activity

Materials

Prerequisite Skills

Activity Outline

Evaluation

Chapter 7

Leisure Activity Categories, Types, and Topics

MS is unpredictable. Some days your loved one may be able to fully participate and enjoy a leisure activity the way they always had, and other days you may have to adapt an activity or the tools used so your loved one can enjoy within their capabilities. As the primary caregiver, you have to decide when assistance is needed. If your loved one is having a flare up, the benefits of activities discussed earlier in this book become even more important. Here are some tips to help you engage your loved one in leisure activities you can both enjoy.

Environment Preparation

Provide sufficient light throughout the room and additional task lighting near the activity when necessary. The area of activity should be lit according to the individual's preferences. The room must also be well lit to eliminate shadows.

Activity Categories

Activities are generally broken down into three different categories: Maintenance Activities, Supportive Activities, and Empowering Activities.

Maintenance Activities

Maintenance activities are traditional activities that help your loved one maintain physical, cognitive, social, spiritual, and emotional health. Examples include:

- Using manipulative games, such as those from R.O.S. Therapy Systems
- Craft and art activities
- Attending church services
- Working trivia and crossword puzzles like the R.O.S. *How Much*

Do You Know About puzzle series
in Amazon or the R.O.S. Store

- Taking a walk

Supportive Activities

Supportive activities are for those that have
a lower tolerance for traditional activities.
These types of activities provide a comfortable
environment while providing stimulation
or solace. Examples include:

- Listening to and singing music
- Hand massages
- Relaxation act'vities, such as
  aromatherapy, meditation, and
  bird-watching

Empowering Activities

Empowering activities help your loved one
attain self-respect by receiving opportunities
for self-expression and responsibility.
Examples include:

- Cooking
- Making memory boxes
- Folding laundry

Activity Types

Once you have chosen an activity from a category that will suit your loved one's need, you must choose an activity type that will interest them. There are several types of activities from which to choose. Below are some examples:

Art Activities

- Coloring
- Mosaic pictures
- Painting
- Dancing

Craft Activities

- Jewelry making
- Holiday centerpieces
- Knitting
- Scrapbooking

Craft Tips:

- ○ Place craft activity supplies in labeled boxes using a broad-tipped black marker.

60

- Group like items for activities together.

- Store materials in different shaped/sized containers or drawers.

- Choose identifying and organizational systems that work best for your loved one.

Verbal Activities

- Conversation
- Trivia

Entertainment Activities

- Board games
- Card games
- Video games
- Crossword puzzles

Crossword Tips:

- Use large-print crossword, word search, or word scramble puzzles. If you cannot find the R.O.S. *How Much Do You Know About* puzzle series or other large-print sources, most copiers have the ability to increase the size of the print so activity items from your local newspaper can be enlarged.

Listening Activities

- Music
- Storytelling
- Books on tape
- Listening to the radio

Visual Activities

- Watching a movie
- Watching a performance
- Watching television

Television Tips: People who are vision impaired or blind do watch television.

○ Adjust the contrast on the TV so colors are either very bright—or only black and white. Adjust in accordance to your loved one's preference.

○ To make the television easier to see, simply turn the screen away from the sun or a lamp so the light source is behind the screen and no glare is shining onto the TV from a light or window.

○ Try moving to a smaller TV, not a larger TV.

Writing Activities

- Writing a story or poem
- Writing a letter

Writing Tips:

○ When additional lighting is necessary, task lighting can be placed in accordance to what is most visually helpful. Table lamps offering the ability to adjust positioning are most helpful in this case.

○ To reduce glare, cover bare lightbulbs of all types with shades. Soften bright light from windows with coverings like blinds or sheer curtains.

○ To help reduce glare and shadowing, position the chair and table so any natural light is behind your loved one versus facing it directly.

○ To prevent shadows, place lamps on the opposite side of the hand being used. Locate bottom edge of lampshade just below eye level.

○ Shiny paper can increase glare. Use matte paper when reading or writing.

Activity Topics

Once you know what category of activity you want to engage your loved one from, here are some suggestions for topics the activity can be based on:

Colors

- Colors of their favorite sports team
- Colors of their wedding
- Colors of flowers or cars

Music

- Favorite music
- Karaoke
- Music from when they were younger and dating
- Patriotic songs
- Holiday songs
- Favorite artists from the age they think they are, e.g., if they believe they are 25 years old, use popular singers or songs of that era.

Military Service

- War stories
- World events of their time
- Their personal experiences of either military service or what it was like in the States

Holidays

- Specific holidays that coincide with their culture or religion
- Favorite holidays

Cooking

- Home cooking
- Comfort food
- Favorite recipes from their mother/grandmother
- Favorite food associated with events, holidays, family gatherings

Sports

- Professional sports teams they liked
- Their involvement in sports
- Big sporting events from their era

School Days

- Where they went to school
- Favorite school classes or teachers
- Sports they played in school
- First kiss
- Memories of their children's school events

Old Cars

- Their family's first car
- Their first car
- Prices of cars now and then
- Dream cars

Places

- Where they were born
- Where they grew up
- Places they have been
- Vacations they took

Chapter 8

Activities of Daily Living
Tips and Suggestions

As we discussed earlier, someone with MS will experience attacks and remissions. They will lose abilities and then partially or fully recover abilities. One day your loved one can dress themselves—the next day they may not be able to. As the primary caregiver, you have to take, and then give back, responsibility for various tasks all the time, especially Activities of Daily Living.

Unlike leisure activities, the Activities of Daily Living discussed in this book are those activities that are a necessary part of everyday life. The following pages contain tips and suggestions for you to use with your loved one.

Bathing

Bathing can be a relaxing, enjoyable experience—or a time of confrontation and anger. Use a calm approach when performing this activity. Maintaining your loved one's "usual" routine is very important.

Safety

- Water temperature should range from 110–115 degrees Fahrenheit maximum to prevent burning or skin injury. Use your elbow to check water temperature.

- The floor of the tub needs to be slip resistant. Use a rubber mat that does not slide, or use permanent nonslip decals.

- Place a nonskid rug on the floor outside the tub to prevent slipping.

- Install grab bars. Always make sure the grab bars are properly and securely installed into the wall studs.

- Do not use bath oils.

- Keep a bell close-by should your loved one need your attention. (MS can cause speech impediments.)

Bathing—Know Your Loved One

- Is your loved one accustomed to a bath or shower?

- Do they, or do they not, need assistance to get into the bath or shower?

- Who is your loved one the most comfortable with when bathing? Is it a female or a male—or a specific caregiver?

*Note: The sex and age of the caregiver can be a significant issue. For example, a 70-year-old female might be upset if a 20-year-old male family member came into the bathroom to assist with care. If your loved one suffers from any emotional symptoms/cognitive impairments associated with MS, their reaction to this caregiver can range from simple embarrassment to fear for their own safety.

Bathing—Communicating and Motivating

If you have to help a loved one bathe:

- Allow your loved one to do what is within their control.

- Stay friendly and respectful.

- Try to avoid arguments by offering a combination of visual cues, step-by-step setup, and short verbal cues.

Bathing—Customary Routines and Preferences

- What time of day does your loved one normally bathe?

- How often did your loved one bathe before MS?

- What is the process that works for you and your loved one when it is time to bathe? Make sure all caregivers know each detail of the process.

For example, is the water turned on and running prior to your loved one entering the tub? Is a towel placed on a shower chair that your loved one may use so that the chill on his or her bottom is removed when sitting?

- Whatever the process, take it one step at a time, following your loved one's normal bathing routine. For example, your loved one may prefer that you wash their hair first and then their body. If sitting in the tub, they may like to soak for 10 minutes before washing.

- Be sure to have your loved one's favorite personal care products for familiar smell and feeling.

Bathing—Planning and Executing

- Use the process that works for the caregiver and loved one when it is time to bathe.

- When your loved one needs assistance undressing, what sequence do they follow to undress? Do they routinely remove their shirt first, followed by their pants, socks, and underwear?

- It can be awkward waiting and watching someone perform such a personal task. As the caregiver, you can provide supervision, but be involved in another activity within the space. For instance, getting towels out while your loved one is undressing is an effective use of the time. Washing your loved one's lower body while they wash their upper body can deflect this discomfort. This also creates a sense of support versus a feeling of total dependence.

- Provide privacy—close blinds, curtains, and doors.

- Ensure your loved one is comfortable. The tub may have a built-in seat, or you may be utilizing a bath/shower chair.

Consider placing a towel on the seat prior because the surface of either is cold against your loved one's skin.

- Avoid drafts and overexposure. Once seated for the bath/shower, your loved one may need a towel draped over their shoulders so they feel less exposed during bathing.

- Have all care items and tools ready prior to beginning.

- Utilize a bath/shower chair if necessary.

- If possible, use a handheld hose for showering and bathing.

- To encourage independence when possible, a long-handled sponge or scrubbing brush can be used if your loved one can scrub themselves.

- Have sponges with soap inside, a soft soap applicator, or a pump bottle with bath soap instead of bar soap. Bar soap can easily slip out of your loved one's hand.

- Remember to **_STOP_** and try another time if your loved one becomes angry or combative.

- Have a towel and clothing prepared for when the bath is finished.

- Use a terry cloth robe instead of a towel to dry off. Always pat the skin dry, avoid rubbing.

Other Bathroom & Grooming Activities

Encourage loved ones to maintain personal grooming habits. Your loved one may need physical or cognitive assistance or both. If your loved one has participated in occupational therapy, utilize the adaptive and compensatory strategies and tips from rehabilitation for optimum independence. For example, you may need to set up the space so that bathing items are easy to reach, adjust shower seating, or use a handheld shower, a checklist for the steps of the task, or teamwork for the hardest parts of the task.

It can sometimes be easier to "do things" for the loved one to save time and mess. In the long run, this serves to make your loved one more dependent.

- Allow plenty of time for routines. If having your loved one do everything independently takes more time than available, select two to four tasks that are most important. Keep in mind the big picture. Your loved one may value being outdoors, volunteering, or exercising more. If time is a factor, save time in personal care routines, and spend time on the activities that bring your loved one the most satisfaction.

- Having someone brush your loved one's teeth is not always a comfortable feeling. Always allow him or her to do what is possible. Adaptive grips might help for holding onto the toothbrush. Electric brushes can compensate for fine motor deficits and often include a timer indicating how long to brush.

- Remember "gently leading" is the best approach. Provide step-by-step directions. This may not be as simple as you think. Stop and think of all of the steps necessary to brush your teeth. From walking into the bathroom, to finding the toothpaste in the drawer and removing the cap, to rinsing their mouth after they have finished brushing. Depending on your loved one's level of cognitive function in association to the MS, it might be easier to show them and have them follow your lead. Family members at home can brush their teeth at the same time.

- Maintaining oral hygiene is very important for those who can no longer do it themselves—or do it thoroughly. Poor hygiene can lead to additional health problems including gum disease, mouth sores, and infections.

Shaving

- Encourage a male to shave if their level of ability allows.
- Use an electric razor for safety.
- Provide assistance if necessary.
- Give positive feedback, and do not verbally correct.

Makeup

- If your loved one had been accustomed to wearing makeup, there is no reason for this to stop. If they show interest or desire to wear makeup, encourage them to do so and offer assistance to apply if needed.

Hair

- Try to maintain hairstyle and care as your loved one did.

- Explain each step simply beforehand to reduce any anxiety. Keep the task as pleasant as possible.

- When washing hair, use nonstinging shampoo. Investigate dry shampoo products.

- Use warm water for washing and rinsing. Tell your loved one before you rinse their hair. The sudden rush of water might be startling.

Nails

- Keep nails clean and trimmed. Be gentle while trimming your loved one's nails. Be mindful of how you pull and where you place their fingers and arms.

- If your loved one had a normal/weekly schedule for nail care prior to MS, please try to maintain that schedule.

- Offer to polish your loved one's nails.

- When polishing, engage your loved one in conversation.

- Avoid trimming toenails—utilize a podiatrist when possible.

Toileting or Using the Bathroom

- Learn your loved one's individual habits and routines for using the toilet. Acknowledge that disease progression or other factors might influence and change your loved one's toileting habits.

- Encourage toileting on rising, before and after meals, and at bedtime at minimum.

- If your loved one is having difficulty with communication, please observe for signs of agitation—pulling at their clothes or walking/pacing restlessly. This may indicate they need to use the bathroom.

- Assist with clothing as needed. Be positive and pleasant while assisting.

- Provide verbal cues and instructions as needed. Be "gently guiding," not controlling or demanding.

Clothing

Clothing—Know Your Loved One

- Initially, clothing choices should remain as they had been and based on your loved one's available wardrobe.

- If personal care is a challenge, clothes need to be comfortable and easy to remove, especially to go to bathroom.

- Choose clothes that are loose fitting and have elastic waistbands.

- If possible, choose clothing that opens in the front, not the back. This prevents your loved one from having to reach behind the body and allows the feeling of independence from dressing one's self.

- For those individuals with motor deficits, when purchasing new clothes, look for clothing with large, flat buttons; Velcro closures; or zippers.

- To assist your loved one with zipping pants or a jacket, attach a zipper pull or leather loop on the end of the zipper.

- If bending and tying shoes is problematic, consider slip-on shoes.

Clothing—Routines and Preferences

- If your loved one has trouble paying attention and making choices, you may have to limit the choice of clothing, and leave only two outfit options in the room at a time.

- If your loved one wants to wear the same thing every day, and if you can afford it, buy three or four sets of the same clothing.

Clothing—Planning and Executing

- Clothes should be laid out according to what goes on first.

- Avoid clothes that are most difficult for your loved one—such as panty hose, knee-high nylons, tight socks, or high heels.

- Make sure that items are not inside out and that buttons, zips, and fasteners are all undone before handing the clothes to your loved one.

Dressing and Undressing

Dressing—Know Your Loved One

Your loved one may just need verbal cues and instructions on dressing. Please remember to allow independent dressing as much as possible to foster an ongoing sense of dignity and independence. As the primary caregiver, you will have to be the judge as to when all caregivers need to begin assisting your loved one with dressing.

Dressing—Communicating and Motivating

- Use short, simple sentences, and provide instruction as needed.

- If your loved one experiences an inability to sustain attention, give instructions in very short steps, such as, "Now put your arm through the sleeve." It may help to use actions to demonstrate these instructions.

- Remember to inquire about going to the toilet before getting dressed.

- Avoid "hovering" while your loved one is dressing. You need to be available as needed during the process, but you can do something like make the bed or straighten up so your loved one does not feel so slow, incompetent, or that you are waiting on them.

Dressing—Routines and Preferences

If you must help your loved one to get dressed, here are some tips:

- Does your loved one get dressed first thing in the morning—before breakfast or after breakfast?

- Does your loved one change into pajamas right before bed—or after dinner?

- Try to maintain your loved one's preferred routine for as long as possible.

- Little things matter. For example, your loved one may like to put on all underwear before putting on anything else.

Dressing—Planning and Executing

- Think about privacy. Make sure that blinds or curtains are closed and that no one will walk in and disturb your loved one while dressing.

If mistakes are made—for example, by putting something on the wrong way—be tactful, or find a way for both of you to laugh about it.

Meals

General Information

- Limit distractions. Serve meals in quiet surroundings, away from the television and other activities. Be sure to have your loved one sit with the sunlight behind them to avoid glare.

- Your loved one might not be able to tell if something is too hot to eat or drink. Always test the temperature of foods and beverages before serving.

- Keep long-standing personal preferences in mind when preparing food. **_However_**, be aware that your loved one may suddenly develop new food preferences or reject foods that were liked in the past.

- Allow your loved one plenty of time to eat. It may take an hour or longer to finish a snack or meal.

- Make meals an enjoyable social event so everyone looks forward to the experience.

- Evaluate your loved one's level of independence, and encourage them to participate at levels that provide success.

Meals—Know Your Loved One

- Can your loved one feed themselves?

- Does your loved one have a visual impairment that may affect their ability to see their meal or drink?

  *Note: As individuals age, they tend to perceive bright, deep colors as lighter. They are able to see yellow, orange, and red more easily than darker colors. Due to normal age-related changes in eyesight, eating and dining may offer additional challenges.

Meals—Communicating and Motivating

- Use short, simple sentences.

- Provide verbal cues/instructions as needed. Remember to be "gently guiding."

- Give your loved one your full attention. Provide direct eye contact.
- Always smile, talk calmly and gently.
- Do not argue, or try to explain "why."

Meals—Routines and Preferences

- No matter what time of day breakfast, lunch, and dinner are served, be consistent every day.
- Offer snacks throughout the day.
- Does your loved one eat their meals at the kitchen table, bedside, or dining room table?
- Factor the length of time it takes your loved one to finish snacks and meals into the overall schedule of the day.

Meals—Planning and Executing

Eating a meal can be a challenge for your loved one with MS, especially if accompanied by declining cognitive function. There are several areas that need to be considered, e.g., visual impairment, physical ailments, and changes in food preferences and dietary restrictions. Here are some simple techniques that can help reduce mealtime problems:

Meal Preparation for MS with Mild Cognitive Deficit Symptoms

- If your loved one wants to assist in making a meal:
  - Make sure cabinets are organized with each item labeled with large easy-to-see labels.
  - Use simple step-by-step written or verbal instructions.
  - You or another caregiver should perform tasks utilizing knives or operating the stove and/or oven.
  - When using a stove top, use the back burners, and turn the pot handles inward toward the back of the stove to avoid any potential grabbing of the pots or pans.

- If for some reason you are not there to supervise:

  - Avoid meals that require the use of the stove. Your loved one may not remember to turn off the stove. They may not be able to distinguish between a pot that is hot or cold.

  - Lay out the ingredients of a meal on the counter or in the refrigerator in labeled containers. Place them in the order that your loved one will use them (similar to laying out their clothes at night).

  - Transfer bulk items, including milk, from a larger container to a smaller container that is easier to lift and pour.

Appropriate Lighting and Eyesight

- Reduce glare by having your loved one sit with the sunlight behind them when eating.

- Use lighting that illuminates the entire dining space and makes objects visible, as well as reducing shadows or reflections.

- Adjust lighting above the table to help see as much detail as possible.

Setting the Table and Serving

- Set each place setting the same way for every meal. Set it the way your loved one is used to, and provide the opportunity to assist in setting the table.

- Decide how to set the rest of the table— main dish, side dishes, seasonings, and condiments. Do it the same way each day. Learn if you will be serving food "family style" or "buffet style." Know your loved one's routines and preferences.

- When pouring a light-colored drink, such as milk, use a dark glass.

- When pouring a dark-colored drink, such as cola, use a white glass.

- Avoid clear glasses. They can disappear from view.

- Use white dishes when eating dark-colored food, and use dark dishes when eating light-colored food.

- To make dishes easier to find on the table, use a tablecloth or placemats that are the opposite color of the dishes.

- Fiesta ware brand dishes have colors (yellow/tangerine) that contrast with most foods so they can be easily seen and will enhance visual perception.

- There should be a clear visual distinction between the table, the dishes, and the food.

- Use solid colors with no distracting patterns.

Eating

This simple, everyday activity requires more maneuvering of objects for someone who is visually impaired. Your loved one may need to develop techniques for items a sighted person may take for granted. Examples include:

"Center Out to Edges" Technique

- Buttering Bread
  - ○ If your loved one can't see how much butter is on a butter dish, help them explore by sliding the knife lightly across the top of the butter to get an idea of where to cut into it.
  - ○ Help your loved one put the piece of butter in the center of the bread, and spread the butter out to the edges of the bread.

The same "center out to edges" technique works equally well for anything of spreadable consistency, making it easier to prepare a sandwich or even ice a cake.

Seasoning Food

- Salt and Pepper
  - Instead of shaking salt and pepper directly onto the food, suggest that your loved one shake it into the palm their hand.
  - Have your loved one pinch and sprinkle the salt and pepper over the food and then taste it.
  - Have your loved one add more salt and pepper in small increments until they have just the right amount.

- Condiments

  The above techniques can be adapted to condiments like ketchup and mustard by placing them to one side of your loved one's plate rather than directly on the food.

  The above techniques can be adapted to liquid seasonings, such as soy sauce or salad dressing—put them in a separate dish and add to the food using a spoon.

94

Cutting Meat

- Have your loved one locate one edge of the meat with the knife and keep the knife there.

- Have your loved one place the fork into the steak about a half-inch from the edge.

- Starting at the edge, have your loved one cut a small semicircle around the fork.

- Encourage your loved one to keep the knife at the edge of the meat while they eat each cut piece.

- Help your loved one repeat the process, and with very little practice it will become automatic.

It is completely appropriate to ask if your loved one would like any assistance.

Chapter 9

Home Preparation

You and your loved one need to feel comfortable, capable, and safe in your home. As the Four Pillars of Engagement are the foundation for all activities, preparation of your home is crucial.

General Organization and Environment

When organizing your loved one's environment, be sure to do it **_with_** them, not for them. Label drawers and cabinets and make sure there is easy access to a phone. The following are general tips that caregivers and family members can use to prepare the home to accommodate your loved one's needs. Decide what works for you and your loved one.

Home Safety Checklist: Bedroom

Issue	Y/N	Options
Lighting Is lighting adequate?		Add light-sensored night-light. Place touch lamp on nightstand. Place rope lighting along hallway leading to bathroom.
Room Clutter Is there too much furniture, too many extra pillows, or too many "stacks of stuff"?		Remove ALL extra furnishings and unnecessary "stacks of stuff." Leave favorite items.
Furniture Clutter Are dresser and nightstand cluttered?		Remove ALL items from nightstand that are not functional and needed. Leave the following items: lamp, phone, plastic drinking glass with top and straw, place for reading glasses and hearing aids. Remove ALL unnecessary items from top of dresser to avoid confusion. Remove unnecessary items and box for storage, donation, or disposal.

Home Safety Checklist: Bedroom

Issue	Y/N	Options
Tripping Hazards Are there tripping hazards?		Remove all throw and scatter rugs. Fix or replace loose floorboards.
Are there rugs or carpets that can be tripped on?		Have professionals restretch loose carpeting to remove lumps and ridges if needed.
Are cords from lamps, TV, or radio out of the way?		Move cords out of walking area. Bundle cords together and attach to baseboards or behind furniture.
Are pathways clear?		Remove any loose items from floor or pathway from room. Organize and box for proper storage, donation, or disposal.
Is there enough room for walking aids?		Make pathway wide enough to accommodate people, wheelchairs, and walking aids.
Furniture Is furniture sturdy enough to provide support if needed?		Antique bedside tables should be replaced with sturdy nightstands.
		If possible, there should be a chair with sturdy arms and legs that is the same height as the bed.
Is bed a sensible height to get into and out of?		Sensible height is if person's thighs are parallel to the floor and feet are flat on the floor when seated on edge of the bed.
		Change out decorative bed frame for a practical bed frame if necessary.

Home Safety Checklist: Bedroom

Issue	Y/N	Options
Bedding		
Is it sensible and practical? Is it too heavy to be moved easily?		Without removing your loved one's favorite blanket, lighten covers as much as possible.
Is there an electric blanket or heating pad?		Never use electric blankets or electric mattress pads.
		Only use heating pads in chairs and never use for extended sleeping hours.

Home Safety Checklist: Closets

Issue	Y/N	Options
Lighting		
Is lighting adequate?		Install task lighting if needed.
Is light pull chain easily accessible?		If possible, change pull chain light fixture to light fixture with switch.
Shelving		
Are shelves easy to reach?		Shelving should be located at a height that person using it can reach items without stretching.
Are shelves original from builder?		Consider removing original shelving from builder and replacing with new, easier-access shelves.
Shoes		
Can shoes be reached without bending over?		If bending is an issue, consider installing an over-the-door shoe rack.
Clothing		
Is closet full of clothing that is no longer being worn?		Never remove your loved one's favorite outfit. Remove unworn or worn out clothing. Leave choices that are easy to match. Keep clothes that are easy to put on and take off.
Are shelves stuffed with a hodgepodge of items that may tumble and fall?		Resolve shelving issue by removing unneeded items and organizing items to box and store, donate, or dispose of.

Home Safety Checklist: Bathroom

Issue	Y/N	Options
Lighting Is lighting adequate? Is light switch easily accessible?		Install task lighting if needed. Change pull chain light to light with switch if possible.
Color Contrast Is the bathroom all white or light colors?		Change wall color so it contrasts with fixtures and counters.
Toilet Is toilet at a height that allows your loved one to sit and stand comfortably?		If possible, add a seat riser or a 3-in-1 commode over the toilet. If possible, replace toilet with a taller model. If possible, install grab bars on both sides at an angle that best suits person who needs them the most.
Mirror Is mirror positioned for sitting and standing? Does mirror cause fear or confusion?		Mirrors may need to be covered or removed for those with dementia as the person may no longer recognize themselves. Mirrors can be removed or covered with a window shade that can be raised or lowered.
Floor Mats and Rugs Is the bathroom floor all white or light colors?		Use rug that is secured with double-sided tape or non-skid padding. Don't use a dark rug—a person with dementia may mistake a dark rug for a hole in the floor.

Home Safety Checklist: Bathroom

Issue	Y/N	Options
Additional Seating Is the bathroom large enough for a chair?		Use a chair in the bathroom to help your loved one while drying themselves after bath or to rest as needed.
Temperature Is the bathroom warm enough?		Some people may get cold easily and need the bathroom warmer than others. A portable heater could be used to warm the bathroom prior to use, but heater should be removed before using the bathroom.
Tub/Shower Does tub/shower have decorative glass doors?		Remove glass doors and replace with a shower curtain.
Are faucets clearly marked *Hot* and *Cold*?		Replace or remark *Hot* and *Cold* faucets.
Are shampoos, conditioners, and soaps in pump dispensers?		Pump dispensers are easier to use than bottles that must be squeezed and/or turned upside down to dispense.
Is there a shower chair available?		Showers can be exhausting. Using a shower chair to rest can help prevent someone from becoming too weak and falling during the shower.
Grab Bars Are there grab bars to make getting into and out of tub or shower easier?		Grab bars should be installed properly and securely into wall studs – not just into tile or fiberglass. Avoid use of suction cups as they can be unreliable.

Home Safety Checklist: Halls and Stairs

Issue	Y/N	Options
Lighting Is lighting adequate?		Use a plug-in night-light. Install light switches on both ends of hallway.
Obstacles Are there obstacles or clutter in hallway?		Remove ALL clutter. Organize and box for proper storage, donation, or disposal—no matter what the item is.
Are there loose floorboards or rugs in hallway?		Repair all loose floorboards. Remove all throw rugs.
Is there furniture in hallway?		Remove all furniture.
Are there doors in hallway?		Keep all doors closed at all times.
Smoke/Carbon Monoxide Detectors Are carbon monoxide and smoke detectors installed?		Install working units on all levels. Replace batteries semiannually.
Handrails Are there handrails in hallway and stairwell?		Install handrails on both sides of hallway and stairwell or secure existing rails.
Stairs Are steps easily seen?		Use neon striping, paint, or duct tape to mark edges of stairs.
Walkers Are walkers easily accessible and transportable?		If possible, keep separate walkers at top and bottom of stairs.

Home Safety Checklist: Kitchen

Issue	Y/N	Options
Lighting Is lighting bright and adequate?		Add task lighting as needed. Bright lights should be located in ceiling above table, countertops, sinks, stove, and in pantry.
Smoke/Carbon Monoxide Detectors Are carbon monoxide and smoke detectors installed?		Install detectors in kitchen. Replace batteries semiannually.
Fire Extinguisher Is there a fire extinguisher in the kitchen?		Make sure fire extinguisher is usable and accessible.
Appliances and their Cords Are there appliances in the kitchen that your loved one cannot or should not use? Are there appliance cords that pose a danger?		Remove appliances that should not or cannot be operated by your loved one on their own. Make sure cords are not near sink or stove.
Counter Clutter Are kitchen counters cluttered?		Keep kitchen counters free of clutter that might cause confusion.
Kitchen Floor Is floor free of tripping hazards?		Remove all rugs, pet food bowls, cords, plants, or any other potential tripping hazards.
Labels Are things visibly and legibly labeled?		Create large-print labels for all switches and containers.

Home Safety Checklist: Kitchen		
Issue	Y/N	Options
Cabinets		
Are doorknobs and cabinet handles easy to use?		Label all cabinets and drawers, and replace difficult-to-use handles, pulls, or knobs.
Are the most-used items within easy reach?		Rearrange cabinets if needed to make the most-used items easiest to reach. Get long-handled grabbers if needed.
Is assistance required to open jars and cans?		Find adaptive tools that work best for your loved one.
Stove		
Does it work properly?		Make sure oven door and burner controls are easy to use and work properly.
Is it easy to use?		Label burners and knobs/controls.
		Clear all items on counters near stove.
Should it be used?		If your loved one has a cognitive issue and shows signs of improper stove use, the caregiver must decide to unplug/disconnect the stove.
		Improper use can be things like: placing items on top of burners forgetting something is cooking forgetting that stove or oven is hot
Microwave Oven		
Does your loved one know what it is and how to use it?		Remove or unplug unit if needed.

Home Safety Checklist: Kitchen

Issue	Y/N	Options
Medication Are medications kept in the kitchen?		Designate a cabinet for your loved one's medication. If more than one person in home takes medication, use separate cabinets.
Step Stools Should a step stool be used?		Step stools can be a hazard and must not be used to reach items that are too high. Find an alternative to a stool if items cannot be stored within person's reach.
Refrigerator Is the food inside still good? Is the food inside covered and stored properly? Is a list of emergency contacts readily available on door?		Designate someone to throw out old or rotten food. The person you are caring for may not know the difference. All food in refrigerator and freezer should be tightly covered and stored properly with a label including what it is and date it was stored. Do not store food on top of refrigerator—out of sight, out of mind! Make sure emergency contact list and information is readily available in "File of Life" pouch on refrigerator door.

Home Safety Checklist: Living Area

Issue	Y/N	Options
Lighting Is lighting adequate?		Room should be evenly lit throughout. Use task lighting and touch lamps as needed.
Flooring and Rugs Is the flooring free of clutter and tripping hazards?		Remove and replace loose floorboards. Area rugs are tripping hazards and should be removed. If floor is carpeted, make sure it has been stretched properly, and ensure there are no lumps or ridges.
Obstacles What are the obstacles in the room?		Remove ALL clutter. Organize and box for proper storage, donation, or disposal—no matter what the item is.
Is there excess furniture?		Remove unnecessary furniture.
Is there room to navigate?		Allow 5½ feet in between each piece of furniture to accommodate use of a wheelchair.
Are there doors in the room?		Keep all doors closed at all times.
Tables Are there glass-topped tables?		Remove all furniture with glass tops.

Home Safety Checklist: Living Area

Issue	Y/N	Options
Tables and Shelving Are tables and shelves full of clutter?		Remove excess clutter from tables and shelves. Organize and box items for proper storage, disposal, or donation.
Chairs and Seating Is the seating comfortable and easy to use?		Use chairs with straight backs, armrests, and firm seats. Make sure seating is a sensible height. Sensible height is if person's thighs are parallel to floor and feet are flat on the floor when seated on the edge of the chair. If needed and possible, add firm cushion to existing pieces to add height. This will make it easier for your loved one to sit down and get up.
Mirrors Does mirror cause fear or confusion?		Mirrors may need to be covered or removed for those with dementia as the person may no longer recognize themselves. Mirrors can be removed or covered with a window shade that can be raised or lowered.
Cords Do they pose a tripping hazard?		Use extension cords sparingly. Secure to baseboards to move them out of the way and prevent tripping.

Home Safety Checklist: Laundry

Issue	Y/N	Options
Lighting Is lighting adequate?		Room should be bright. Add lighting as needed.
Clutter and Organization Is room free of tripping hazards?		If possible, find a place—other than on the floor—to store laundry basket. Remove all unnecessary items and box for proper storage, donation, or disposal.
Supplies Are laundry supplies organized and properly labeled? Can laundry supplies be easily reached without stretching?		Organize and label laundry supplies. Ensure laundry supplies are within easy reach.
Washer and Dryer Are washer and dryer easy and convenient to use? Are dryer lint trap and vent hose cleaned regularly?		Washer and dryer should be located side by side so that wet clothes do not have to be moved from room to room. To prevent fires, clean lint trap and vent hose regularly.
Ventilation Is the room well ventilated?		Keep windows and/or doors open when in room for proper ventilation.

Home Safety Checklist: Basement

Issue	Y/N	Options
Stairs		
Are there handrails on both sides of the steps?		Install railings as needed.
Do railings or steps have loose or uneven wood or potential for splinters?		Repair or replace wood that is loose or splintered.
Are items stacked on the steps?		Remove unnecessary items and box for storage, donation, or disposal.
Lighting		
Is lighting adequate?		Basement should be bright. Add lighting as needed.
Are light switches located at top and bottom of stairs?		Install additional switches as needed.
Clutter and Organization		
Is room free of trip hazards?		Remove unnecessary items and box for storage, donation, or disposal.
		If possible, find a place—other than on the floor—to store laundry basket.
Shelving		
Is shelving sturdy enough to hold items placed on it?		Remove unnecessary items and box for storage, donation, or disposal.
Are items on shelves neatly stacked so they will not fall off?		Shelving should be located at a height that person using it can reach items without stretching.
Frequently Used Items		
Are frequently used items within easy reach?		Organize items so that most-used items are easiest to reach.

Home Safety Checklist: Garage

Issue	Y/N	Options
Stairs Are there handrails on both sides of the steps?		Install railings as needed.
Do railings or steps have loose or uneven wood or potential for splinters?		Repair or replace wood that is loose, uneven, or splintered.
Are items stacked on the steps?		Remove unnecessary items and box for storage, donation, or disposal.
Lighting Is lighting adequate?		Garage should be bright. Add lighting as needed.
Are light switches located at top and bottom of stairs?		Install additional switches as needed.
Tools and Equipment Are sharp tools away from walkways and hung or stored properly?		Hang or store sharp tools properly for safety and to prevent tripping hazards.
Is machinery or equipment blocking walkway?		Remove unnecessary items, and box for storage, donation, or disposal.
Are frequently used tools and equipment easily accessible?		Organize space so that most-used items are easily accessible.
Clutter and Organization Is room free of tripping hazards?		Remove unnecessary items and box for storage, donation, or disposal.

Home Safety Checklist: Garage		
Issue	Y/N	Options
Frequently Used Items Are frequently used items easily accessible?		If items are used inside the home, consider storing those items inside. Remove unnecessary items, and box for storage, donation, or disposal.
Garage Door Does garage door have an automatic opener?		Automatic garage door openers make it easier to get in and out of the garage. Check batteries in opener and in the main box semiannually.

Home Safety Checklist: Foyer

Issue	Y/N	Options
Lighting Is lighting sufficient inside foyer and outside on porch?		Add lighting as needed.
Doorbell Can doorbell be heard all throughout home?		Repair or replace doorbell so that it can be heard anywhere in the home.
Door, Window, and Peephole Can you see who is standing on the front porch or stoop?		Clear window or install peephole to be able to identify people before opening the door.
Closet Is coat closet easy to use and not too cluttered? Is there room to store hats, scarves, gloves, and boots?		Remove unnecessary items and box for storage, donation, or disposal. If there is no closet, install sturdy hooks for coats, hats, scarves, and gloves.
Doormat Is there a doormat and is it appropriate?		Use an absorbent mat with a non-skid backing. Don't use a dark mat – a darker mat could be mistaken for a hole in the floor.
Door Can door be easily locked? Is there a dead bolt lock on the door?		If a person is in early stages of dementia, doors should be secured to prevent wandering. Install latches high on door so they cannot be easily reached.

Home Safety Checklist: Porch, Yard, Driveway

Issue	Y/N	Options
Lighting		
Do exterior porch and garage lights illuminate entire areas?		Add lighting or replace bulbs with the highest wattage the fixture allows.
Is yard lighting equipped with motion detectors?		If possible, install motion detector lights for safety and security.
Steps and Rails		
Are there sturdy rails to use for climbing up and down stairs?		Repair or replace rails as needed to ensure proper sturdiness and safety.
Are rails smooth and free of splinters?		Repair or replace rails to prevent injury from cracks or splinters.
Are there any loose or wobbly steps?		Repair or replace any loose or wobbly steps to prevent trip/fall hazard.
Are steps slippery in wet conditions?		Add non-slip material to stair treads to prevent them from becoming slippery when wet.
Sidewalks and Driveway		
Do sidewalks and driveway have cracks or loose cement that could be trip hazards?		Repair any cracks or loose cement that could be potential trip hazards. Be aware of tree roots that may affect paved surfaces.
Mailbox		
Is there a clear path to the mailbox?		Make arrangements with the Post Office to have mail delivered to door for a person who is elderly or disabled.

Lighting, Glare, and Contrast

Depending on your loved one's eye condition, cognitive deficit, or individual preference, you may find it necessary to modify existing lighting, glare, and contrast in the home. People will not always admit that they have an issue with their vision, but if they do, it will affect their ability to engage in an activity. Here are some tips to help:

Lighting

The following lighting changes could be key in your loved one's safety and ability to perform tasks independently.

- Fluorescent lighting can contribute to an increase in glare. Try different types of bulbs to see which is most comfortable for your loved one.

- Keep all rooms evenly lit and lighting level consistent throughout the house so shadows and dangerous bright spots are eliminated.

- Make sure light switches, pull cords, and lamps are easily accessible for your loved one in case they are in a wheelchair.

- If possible, purchase touch lamps or lamps that can be turned on or off by sound.

- Depending on the individual, additional task lighting may be necessary in certain areas of the home.

Glare

Glare can be caused by sunlight or light from a lamp. Glare can make it difficult for an individual with low vision to see when the glare hits shiny surfaces, including glossy paint on walls. Sunglasses can be beneficial both indoors and outside for someone who is light sensitive.

- Enable sunlight to fill the room with light without producing glare. Adjust sunlight coming from windows by using mini blinds and altering their position throughout the day. If mini blinds are not available, use sheer curtains.

- Be aware when placing mirrors in a room. Mirrors placed across from larger windows can significantly increase the amount of light in a room, but they can also be the source of a significant amount of glare.

- Cover bare lightbulbs of all types with shades.

- Position chairs and tables so that when your loved one is sitting on a chair or at a table, they do not have to look directly at the light coming from the window.

- Cover or remove shiny/reflective surfaces, such as floors and tabletops.

Color Contrasts

Using contrast is a key strategy if your loved one has a visual impairment. The more contrast, the easier it is to find and use objects or activity items around the house.

- Put light-colored objects against a dark background.

- Avoid upholstery with patterns for seated activities. Stripes, plaids, and checks can be visually confusing.

- Opt for solid-colored tables and countertops in a neutral tone. Countertops with busy patterns can make it difficult to locate items and can be more difficult to keep clean.

- In a room with mostly dark tones, place light-colored pillows or chairs in strategic places to help your loved one find things and get around easily.

Chapter 10

Put Your Mask on First

There will be many challenges to you personally in this caregiving journey that can and will wear you down. As a caregiver, first and foremost, you must take care of yourself in order to be able to assist your loved one. That might be easier said than done, but please make every effort to do so. The following are some general tips for you, the family caregiver:

About You

- Put yourself first (this is not being selfish) —if you are not in good physical or mental health you cannot help anyone.
- Arrange some time for yourself.
- Keep a strong support system.
- Do not be afraid to ask for help.
- Keep contact with friends.
- Define priorities; do not try to be all things to all people.

Stress

- Recognize your own stress and take steps to minimize. Stress can be exhibited in multiple ways:
  - Anger
  - Helplessness
  - Embarrassment
  - Grief
  - Depression
  - Isolation
  - Physical illness

Burnout

Burnout for caregivers results from physical and emotional exhaustion.

It is important to realize a family member, spouse, or hired caregiver experiences the same emotions as staff in health care facilities, but may not have the needed support system. Suggestions to avoid burnout:

- Know what makes you angry or impatient. Make a list.

- Look for the reason behind behavior.
- Use relaxation techniques, e.g., deep breathing, imagery, and music.
- Ask for help, and accept help when it is offered!

Caregiving is a challenging road with constant twists and turns, from the change in your role/relationship with your loved one, to dealing with the strains of a 24/7 job of caring for that loved one. As much as you may feel like you are alone, please know that you are not. Millions of family caregivers are dealing with the same issues that you are. Do not be embarrassed to share details about what you are experiencing, and do not be afraid to ask for help. There are individuals, organizations, and support groups throughout the country that are available to you. There is also R.O.S. —we were built on the simple mission of our founder's need to help his mother and father during a 25-year battle with Parkinson's and dementia. We understand what you are going through, and we are here to help.

Personal History Form

This is _____'s Personal History

Name: _____

Maiden Name: _____

Date of Birth: _____

Preferred Name: _____

Name and relationship of people completing this history:

_____

_____

_____

*What age do you think the person thinks they are?

_____

*Do they ask for their spouse but do not recognize them?

_____

*Do they look for their children but do not recognize them? _____

*Do they look for their mom? _____

*Do they perceive themselves as younger? Please describe. _____

_____

Describe the "home" they remember. _____

_____

_____

_____

Describe the person's personality prior to the onset
of multiple sclerosis. _____

_____

_____

What makes the person feel valued? Talents, occupation,
accomplishments, family, etc. _____

_____

_____

What are some favorite items they must always have in
sight or close by? _____

_____

_____

What is their exact morning daily routine? _____

_____

_____

_____

_____

What is their exact evening routine?

_____

_____

_____

_____

What type of clothing do they prefer? Do they like to choose their own clothes for the day, or do they prefer to have their clothes laid out for them?

_____

_____

_____

_____

What is their favorite beverage?

_____

What is their favorite food?

_____

What will get them motivated? (Church, friends coming over, going out, etc.)

_____

_____

_____

_____

List significant interests in their life, such as hobbies, recreational activities, job related skills/experiences, military experience, etc.

- Age 8 to 20:

_____

_____

_____

- Age 20 to 40:

_____

_____

_____

What is their religious background? (Affiliation, prayer time, symbols, traditions, church/synagogue name, etc. Did they lead any services or sing in the choir?)

_____

_____

_____

What type of music do they enjoy listening to, playing, or singing? Do they have any musical talents?

_____

_____

_____

What is their favorite TV program? Movie?

_____

_____

_____

Did they enjoy reading? Which authors, topics, or genres do they prefer? Would they listen to audiobooks or books on tape?

_____

_____

_____

_____

Can they tell the difference between someone on TV and a real person?

_____

_____

Marital status - If married more than once, provide specifics. Include names of spouses, dates of marriage, and other relevant information.

_____

_____

_____

_____

_____

List distinct characteristics about their spouse(s), such as occupations, personality traits, or daily routine.

_____

_____

_____

_____

_____

Do they have children? Be sure to include children both living and deceased. Include names, birth dates, and any other relevant information.

_____

_____

_____

_____

_____

Who do they ask for the most? What is their relationship with this person(s)? Describe how that person typically spends their day.

_____

_____

_____

_____

_____

What causes your loved one stress?

_____

_____

_____

_____

**What calms them down when they are stressed
or agitated?**

_____

_____

_____

_____

**How long has it been since multiple sclerosis symptoms
first appeared?**

_____

**Describe how the symptoms of multiple sclerosis are
affecting your loved one.**

_____

_____

_____

_____

_____

Have they accepted the multiple sclerosis?

_____

_____

What activities do they feel they can no longer participate in as a result of the multiple sclerosis?

_____

_____

_____

_____

What specific activities did they enjoy prior to multiple sclerosis diagnosis?

_____

_____

_____

_____

Are they participating less frequently with family and friends? Can you identify why?

_____

_____

_____

_____

Other information that would help to bring joy to your loved one.

_____

_____

_____

_____

_____

_____

_____

_____

_____

_____

_____

_____

_____

_____

_____

_____

_____

_____

_____

_____

_____

_____

_____

_____

_____

_____

_____

_____

_____

_____

_____

_____

_____

_____

_____

_____

_____

_____

_____

_____

*Note: This form includes questions that are being asked in case your loved one has dementia symptoms in addition to multiple sclerosis.

About the Authors

Scott Silknitter

Scott Silknitter is the founder of R.O.S. Therapy Systems. He designed and created the R.O.S. Play Therapy™ System, the *How Much Do You Know About* Series of themed activity books and the R.O.S. *BIG Book*. Starting with a simple backyard project to help Mom and Dad, Mr. Silknitter has dedicated his life to improving the quality of life for all seniors through meaningful education, entertainment and activities.

Suzanne John, RN

Suzanne John is a retired Registered Nurse. She possesses over 12 years of clinical nursing experience in areas, such as Cardiothoracic Surgical nursing, Medical and Cardiac Intensive Care nursing, working with ventilator-dependent patients and their families in a long-term care facility, Supervising RN in a skilled nursing facility, and as a RN providing outpatient cardiac rehab care to patients post open-heart surgery or after a "heart attack." Suzanne believes, "a nurse should be intelligent in her knowledge of the human body and medicine to practice safe care, but a nurse's success is obtained in her ability to interact and relate to her patient's condition and establish a trusting and respectful relationship." Suzanne currently teaches students studying to earn a caregiver certificate how to perform Activities of Daily Living.

Lisa Ost-Beikmann, ADC, CDP, AC-BC, CADDCT, CAEd

Lisa Ost-Beikmann is the Director of Education for the National Association of Activity Professionals (NAAP), with a nine-year career in Geriatrics and Activities.

Lisa is an active member of the aging care community. She has worked tirelessly to help guide the community through her membership and various roles at the following organizations: Kansas Activity Directors Association (KADA), Kansas Partnership for Improving Dementia Care (KPIDC), National Association of Activity Professionals (NAAP), National Certification Council of Activity Professionals (NCCAP), National Council of Certified Dementia Practitioners (NCCDP), and National Certification Board for Alzheimer's Care (NCBAC).

With a focus on person-centered care and improving quality of life through activities and engagement, Lisa teaches the Alzheimer's Disease and Dementia Care Training course and speaks at multiple state and national events.

References

1. *The Handbook of Theories on Aging* (Bengtson et al., 2009)
2. *Activity Keeps Me Going, Volume 1* (Peckham et al., 2011)
3. *Essentials for the Activity Professional in Long-Term Care* (Lanza, 1997)
4. *Abnormal Psychology*, Butcher
5. www.dhspecialservices.com
6. National Certification Council for Dementia Practitioners www.NCCDP.org
7. "Managing Difficult Dementia Behaviors: An A-B-C Approach" By Carrie Steckl
8. Iowa Geriatric Education Center website, Marianne Smith, PhD, ARNP, BC Assistant Professor University of Iowa College of Nursing
9. *Excerpts taken from "Behavior...Whose Problem is it?" Hommel, 2012
10. *Merriam-Webster's Dictionary*
11. "The Latent Kin Matrix" (Riley, 1983)
12. *Care Planning Cookbook* (Nolta et al.2007)
13. "Long-Term Care" (Blasko et al. 2011)
14. "Success Oriented Programs for the Dementia Client" (Worsley et al 2005)
15. Heerema, Esther. "Eight Reasons Why Meaningful Activities Are Important for People with Dementia." www.about.com
16. *Activities 101 for the Family Caregiver* (Appler-Worsley, Bradshaw, Silknitter)
17. American Foundation for the Blind
18. www.aging.com
19. www.WebMD.com
20. www.nlm.nih.gov
21. www.caregiver.org
22. www.nationalmssociety.org
23. *Textbook of Medical-Surgical Nursing*, Brunner/Suddarth, 5th edition

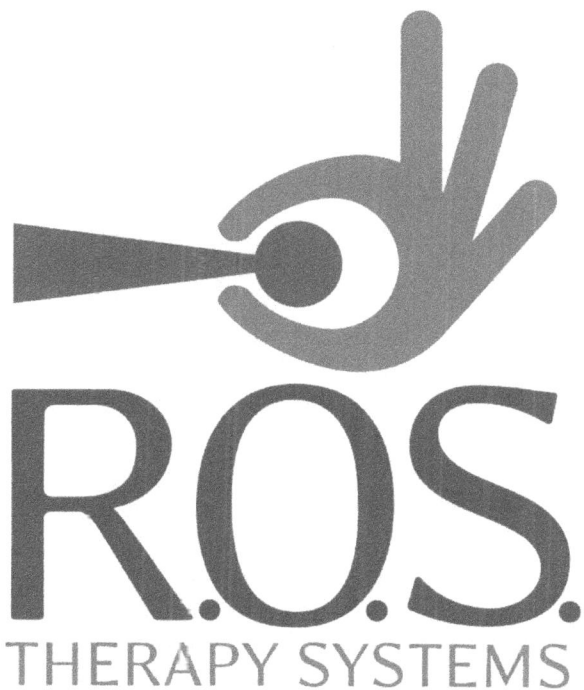

R.O.S.
THERAPY SYSTEMS

For additional assistance, please contact us at:
www.ROSTherapySystems.com
888-352-9788